Sweet Wellness

LEADING A SUGAR-WISE LIFESTYLE

ONEN JOSHUA

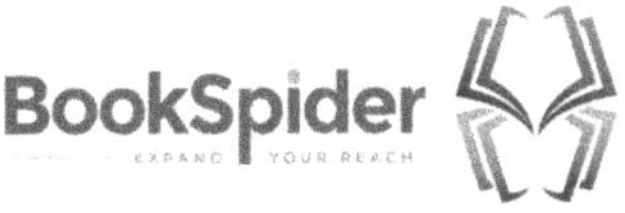

ISBN:

Published by **BookSpider**

No. 16, Olubunmi Johnson, Fagbile Estate,
Isolo-Ijegun Way, Lagos, Nigeria.

Phone line: +234 816 056 0570

hello@bookspider.ng

www.bookspider.ng

DEDICATION

This book is dedicated to anyone who seeks to live a life of sweet wellness.

It is dedicated to those who are committed to their health and well-being and are willing to embark on a transformative journey towards a sugar-smart lifestyle.

It is also dedicated to those who have faced challenges, setbacks, and moments of doubt yet remain resilient in their pursuit of balance and vitality; those who have supported and inspired others on their sugar-smart journeys, thus creating a community of empowerment and encouragement, those who believe in the power of mindfulness, self-care and making mindful choices that nurture both the body and the soul.

May this book serve as a beacon of knowledge, inspiration, and guidance as you navigate the path toward optimal health, mindfulness, and a life filled with sweetness and well-being.

TABLE OF CONTENTS

ACKNOWLEDGEMENTS

I want to express my heartfelt gratitude to all those who have contributed to creating this book, *Sweet Wellness: Leading a Sugar-Wise Lifestyle.* Their support, guidance, and expertise have been invaluable in bringing this project to life.

I thank my family and loved ones for their unwavering encouragement throughout the book-writing phase. Their understanding of the importance of a healthy life and their utmost belief in my pursuits continue to inspire me.

My deepest appreciation goes to the researchers, authors, and health professionals whose work shaped my understanding of the impact of sugar on human health. Their dedication to scientific inquiry and dissemination of knowledge has been instrumental in educating and empowering individuals worldwide.

I also want to thank the nutritionists, dietitians, and wellness experts who provided insights and practical tips through numerous resources. Their expertise and passion for helping others make informed choices have enriched the content of this book.

I am deeply grateful to the team that assisted in making this book a success. I appreciate the beta readers and reviewers who generously shared their feedback and suggestions during the editing process. I also appreciate the publishers, editors, and designers who worked diligently to transform the manuscript into a polished and visually appealing book. The insights, constructive criticism, commitment to excellence, and attention to detail that each person contributed ensured the overall clarity and effectiveness of the book.

Dear reader, thank you for picking up this book. Your curiosity, commitment to personal growth, and willingness to live a healthier life motivated me to create a resource that can make a positive impact on your journey.

By applying the strategies explored in this book, I believe we can all create a world where a balanced lifestyle and informed decision-making prevail. Thank you for your unwavering support and belief in the power of leading a sugar-smart lifestyle!

With heartfelt gratitude,

Onen Joshua

INTRODUCTION

Being healthy requires intentionality.

How often have you heard the phrase, 'You are what you eat?' Let's assume you learnt about it today; how did that realisation make you feel? That the food you consume affects your body significantly. Interesting, right?

While humans consume many foods and edible substances, sugar has always been the one they are weary of. Sugar is many things to us. Whereas there is the white granular substance directly consumed in its raw form in accompaniment with other foods, there's also the by-product of whole foods we consume, which, when fully broken down by our digestive system, turns to sugar. Apparently, humans cannot do without consuming sugar, one way or another.

In a world seemingly fuelled by sugar, it is easy to yield to the irresistible charm of its sweet allure. From mouthwatering desserts to comforting snacks, sugar has seamlessly integrated itself into our daily existence, becoming an indispensable component of our contemporary eating habits. However, beneath its seductive sweetness lies an obscured peril that jeopardises our overall health and vitality. Since we can't entirely do without sugar, how can we consume enough, not too much, to make us function to our strongest capability and still live healthily? That is what I have fleshed out in this book.

Over time, our connection with sugar has undergone a transformation. Sugar used to be considered a rare and precious commodity. But now, it has permeated every aspect of our food industry and daily lives. Unfortunately, this widespread presence has contributed to a multitude of health issues, such as obesity, diabetes, cardiovascular diseases, and various related ailments. As a matter of fact, men are advised to consume less sugar so their sexual game can be top-tier. Women, too, are advised to stay clear of sugary foods if they want to have balanced menstrual health and, thus, less cramps during their periods.

Indeed, sugar is an integral part of human life, irrespective of gender. As a result, the need to reevaluate our consumption decisions, equip ourselves with knowledge, and regain mastery over our well-being has become more urgent than ever before.

At some point in my life, I consumed more sugar than my body needed to function properly. I know you have, as well. How does one escape sugar consumption when tongue-arousing cravings push us to indulge in savoury pleasures? But in whatever way we turn the situation, the fact will remain that staying healthy is an intentional journey that requires cutting down on some things we consume to maintain our health and increase our life span.

This book, therefore, invites you to embark on a transformative journey, guiding you toward a lifestyle that frees you from the clutches of excessive sugar consumption. Whether you're a fervent advocate for conscious eating or someone who's seeking a positive change, this book is your compass to navigate the complex world of nutrition and wellness.

Because this book is intended to take you on a journey, we'll start by exploring the prevalence of sugar in our society today. Understanding the impact of sugary diets on our health and how to conquer sugar cravings to reduce sugar consumption is another important step in leading a sugar-wise lifestyle. Also, there's a role that physical activity plays in helping you break down sugar. The concluding chapters will delve into the steps you can take to nurture and sustain a sugar-wise lifestyle. How you can navigate social situations and challenges, and further resources to aid your commitment to this new lifestyle.

Are you intrigued? Come journey with me through the pages of this book, where I will unravel effective strategies and insights to guide you toward embracing a sugar-wise lifestyle. Together, let us discover the path forward and embark on a transformative journey towards a healthier, more mindful relationship with sugar.

Chapter One

THE BITTERSWEET TEMPTATION

As a busy working professional navigating through your typical day, you begin your morning with a seemingly healthy breakfast of yoghurt and granola, unaware that the flavoured yoghurt contains a high amount of added sugar. As you head to work, you stop by the supermarket to pick up some appetisers. You probably want something to eat while working, so you opt for chin chin.

At lunchtime, you rush to grab a quick meal from a nearby fast-food restaurant, believing you're making a relatively healthy choice with a chicken salad, without realising that your salad's dressing contains hidden sugars. Exhausted after a long day, you crave a convenient dinner option when you arrive home. You opt for a frozen meal, assuming it will save you the stress of preparing a fresh meal. But you must realise that these pre-packaged meals often contain significant amounts of hidden sugars to enhance flavour and prolong shelf life. You can see that throughout the day, your meal choices seemed relatively innocuous, but the truth is that there is a significant amount of sugar in your diet without your knowledge.

The prevalence of added sugars in everyday foods has become a societal norm, leading to various health problems. Excessive sugar consumption results in weight gain, elevated risk of developing chronic illnesses like diabetes and heart disease, and even impacts oral health.

This illustration is a typical example of how sugar has stealthily made its way into the average person's meal choices. It highlights the importance of creating awareness about the hidden sugar epidemic, encouraging individuals to be mindful of the sources and amounts of sugar in their diets.

By making informed food choices, reading labels, and opting for whole, unprocessed foods, individuals can take control of their health and reduce the detrimental effects of excessive sugar consumption in their daily lives.

In a world filled with delectable treats and tantalising flavours, it's hard to resist the allure of sugary delights. Our modern lives are replete with sugary temptations, from candies and cakes to sodas and pastries. Yet, beneath their deceptively enticing exteriors lies a bittersweet truth that we must confront: the consequences of a sugary diet.

The Rise of Sweet Seduction

There is an increase in the prevalence of sugary products that captivate and entice people today. We are constantly bombarded with marketing campaigns that list foods that appeal to our cravings. This raises your longing to choose a specific sugary food. Pampering your cravings can put you at high risk, from having dental health issues to chronic health conditions like diabetes.

The history of our infatuation with sugary foods dates back to centuries. Sugar, once considered a rare and precious commodity, has transformed into a readily available staple in our daily lives. With technological advancements and increased globalisation, sugar has become cheaper and more accessible. It has infiltrated our diets, from breakfast cereals to salad dressings.

But in ancient times, sugar was a luxury good only available to the wealthy due to its scarcity and expensive production costs. Its sweetness and capacity to improve the flavour of food and beverages made it highly prized.

The need for sugar increased over the centuries as trade and exploration routes evolved. Sugar was produced in large quantities, notably in areas like the Caribbean and the Americas, thanks to the growth of colonial plantations and the Transatlantic slave trade. Sugar cane was grown and processed on these plantations using slave labour, which boosted accessibility and cost.

The Industrial Revolution's technological developments significantly revolutionised the sugar industry. Because of innovations like steam-powered mills and refining methods, sugar processing became more productive and cost-effective. However, with industrialisation, sugar stopped being a luxury item for the wealthy and became a common household ingredient.

Growing globalisation and the development of efficient transportation infrastructure facilitated sugar trading on international markets. It arrived in kitchens and on dinner tables worldwide after being transported and disseminated across continents. Due to their availability and natural sweetness, sugary foods have become a common part of our diets.

The amount of sugar in our diets nowadays is unprecedented. It is now available in everyday products, including desserts and sweets. Breakfast cereals, yoghurt, sauces, processed snacks, and even foods like salad dressings that seem healthful have hidden sugars.

Our diets contain a lot of sugar, which raises questions about how it will affect our health. Overindulging in sugar has been connected to dental issues, diabetes, heart disease, and obesity. The attraction and addictive qualities of sugar continue to contribute to its pervasiveness in our daily lives despite growing awareness of these health dangers. Understanding how sugar has changed historically from a rare luxury to a common element helps us better understand how our obsession with sugary foods has changed. In light of this sugary infiltration, it also emphasises how crucial it is to consume food mindfully, read food labels, and make educated decisions to maintain a balanced and healthy diet.

The Sugar Trap

Sugar tastes so good, but why are there warnings to desist from our sweet cravings?

Say you drink tea every day. You scoop in a teaspoon filled with sugar. And you do that for one year. That is how much sugar an average person consumes regularly. The allure of sugar lies in its ability to hijack our taste buds and trigger a cascade of pleasure-inducing chemicals in our brains.

It tantalises our senses, providing a momentary bliss that keeps us returning for more. However, this sweet seduction comes at a cost. Studies have shown that excessive sugar consumption can result in several health issues, such as type 2 diabetes, obesity, heart disease, and tooth decay. It links to mental health issues like depression and anxiety. Sugar is a trap and contains no nutritional value. Every teaspoon or cube of sugar contains about 20 calories. Sugar harms our bodies and only gives us excess calories. Too much sugar intake is converted into fat and deposited in adipose tissue.

One harm sugar brings to our bodies is that we tend to age faster through glycation. There are harmful radicals in sugar called Advanced Glycation End Products (AGEs). Your sugar intake accumulates in your body to damage protein, making you age faster. You notice your skin getting dried quicker and reducing your vision quality. So, save yourself the stress and escape the sugar trap before it captures you.

Hidden Sweeteners

Let's dive into the world of hidden sweeteners. You'd be surprised to learn how cunningly sugar disguises itself in our favourite food products, often adopting names we are unaware of. A few examples of hidden sweeteners lurking in our favourite snacks and beverages are high-fructose corn syrup (HFCs), dextrose, sucrose, and maltose. Even seemingly healthy options, like yoghurt and granola bars, can be loaded with sugars. Unbeknownst to many, our seemingly innocent food choices may contribute to our sugar intake more than we realise. Behind their health-conscious façade, these products can secretly pack a sugary punch, leaving many of us unaware of the extent to which our seemingly innocent food choices contribute to our overall sugar intake.

So, let's play detective and become label-reading pros. We need to unmask the different aliases that sugar hides behind. Watch out for high-fructose corn syrup, that crafty sweetener derived from corn. Then there's dextrose, a simple sugar that plays tricks in various processed foods. Sucrose, the classic table sugar made from sugar cane or beets, often creeps into our diets in ways we least expect. And let's not forget maltose, the sugar derived from grains, slyly appearing in cereals, bread, and malted drinks.

Even products with health claims or targeting specific dietary needs may contain hidden sweeteners. Yoghurt, for instance, can be a stealthy source of sugar, especially flavoured or fruit-infused varieties that rely on added sugars for taste enhancement. Granola bars, often perceived as wholesome and nutritious, can harbour substantial amounts of added sugars disguised by other ingredients or clever marketing tactics.

Understanding the prevalence of hidden sweeteners empowers us to make more informed dietary choices. By scrutinising nutrition labels, looking beyond front-of-package claims, and familiarising ourselves with the various names of added sugars, we can take control of our sugar intake and make healthier decisions.

Remember, knowledge is the key to unravelling the mysteries of hidden sweeteners and promoting a well-balanced and mindful approach to our diet.

Breaking Free from the Sugar Shackles

There is nothing to be ashamed of if you have high-sugar cravings. At some point in our lives, we all craved sugary substances. It only takes some personal discipline to break free from the sugar shackles, as it can be difficult.

One proven method to break free from the sugar trap is asking yourself some valuable questions. Take note of these five valuable questions to ask yourself.

- Am I aware of the frequency and quantity of my sugar intake?

- Am I mindful of the various names sugar can take in food products?

- How do I feel after consuming sugary foods? Do I experience energy crashes, mood swings, or cravings shortly after eating sweets?

- How can I become a more conscious label reader? Am I taking the time to thoroughly examine nutrition labels and ingredient lists to identify hidden sugars in the foods I purchase?

- What strategies can I implement to reduce my sugar intake gradually? Can I start by cutting back on sugary beverages or reducing the amount of added sugar in my favourite recipes?

Acknowledging the impact of a sugary diet is the first step towards reclaiming control over your health. It's time to break free from the sugar shackles and embark on a journey toward a more balanced and mindful approach to eating.

By understanding the detrimental effects of excessive sugar consumption, you can make informed decisions about what you put into your body. With knowledge, willpower, and healthier alternatives, you can gradually reduce your reliance on sugary foods and experience the benefits of a more wholesome diet.

As we conclude this chapter, we now understand the deceptive nature of sugary diets. While their taste may be undeniably tempting, sugar has a detrimental effect on our health, which cannot be ignored. It is within our power to make mindful choices, to be aware of hidden sugars, and to embrace healthier alternatives.

In the following chapters, we will delve deeper into the consequences of sugary diets and explore practical strategies to overcome this bittersweet temptation. Together, we can navigate the world of nutrition and pave the way to a healthier, more balanced life.

Chapter Two

UNMASKING THE SWEET SABOTEURS

In the previous chapter, we uncovered the bittersweet truth about sugary diets and their impact on one's health. Armed with this knowledge, we will be unmasking the sweet saboteurs that stealthily infiltrate our daily lives. I will also highlight how to identify disguised sugar in processed foods and the hidden culprits contributing to excessive sugar consumption, like our sugar-loaded pantries, food labels, and the beverage trap. Finally, we'll explore our emotional connection with sugar and alternative ways to cope with stress, find solace, or celebrate without relying on sugar-loaded snacks. This knowledge will empower you to make informed choices and regain control over your well-being.

What do I mean by unmasking the sweet saboteurs, you may ask? First off, a saboteur deliberately destroys, damages, or obstructs something. In this context, processed foods are the sweet saboteurs because they harbour sugar in the most inconspicuous ways. Your journey to unmasking the sweet saboteurs begins in the heart of your home — from your pantry. Often stocked with convenience foods and snacks, the pantry can harbour a multitude of sugar-laden products that you unwittingly consume. Investigating labels and scrutinising ingredient lists thus becomes essential in identifying the culprits.

Breakfast cereals, flavoured yoghurts, sauces, and even seemingly innocent condiments can be laden with added sugars. Hence, it is time to reassess your pantry choices and replace sugar-heavy options with healthier alternatives to create a supportive environment for your well-being. Even with good meal planning, there will be times when you need to whip up a small meal quickly. Having a pantry stocked with common healthy foods can help you keep your meals simple and healthy.

The Beverage Trap

While we often associate sugary diets with food, it's crucial not to overlook the significant contribution of sugary beverages. Sodas, energy drinks, fruit juices, and even flavoured coffees and teas can harbour shocking amounts of added sugars. We will explore the hidden sugar content in these drinks and their impact on health. By unmasking the sweet saboteurs in your beverage choices, you can opt for healthier alternatives such as water, herbal teas, or freshly squeezed juices to quench your thirst without compromising your well-being.

Hidden Sugars and Their Impact on Health

Hidden sugars are added sugars with less-known names and in products where you would not expect to find them. Now, let's examine the different types of sugars:

- **Naturally-Occurring Sugars**

  These sugars are those (mostly fructose and lactose) found in fruits, dairy, vegetables, and other natural products. They are found in whole foods, so other nutrients like fibre, minerals, vitamins, antioxidants, and water naturally accompany them.

- **Refined Sugars**

  These types of sugars are obtained by extraction from foods like corn, beets, sugarcane, etc. They are often added to processed foods to increase their sweetness.

- **Added Sugars**

  Added sugars, as the name portrays, are sugars and syrups added to food products during production, preparation, processing, or consumption. Typical examples of added sugars include sucrose, glucose, fructose, dextrose, and high-fructose corn syrup.

Below are some of the negative impacts of hidden sugars on our health:

- **High Blood Pressure**

  Consuming too much sugar increases the risk of developing high blood pressure, posing a threat to cardiovascular health.

- **Neuroinflammation**

Sugar consumption has been linked to the risk of causing neuro-inflammation, which can damage the hippocampus, leading to memory problems and difficulties with spatial orientation.

- **Cavity**

Sugar serves as a food source for bacteria in the mouth, which then produce acid. This acid attacks the teeth, leading to cavities and other dental issues.

- **Hyperglycemia**

Excessive sugar consumption can result in hyperglycemia, damaging the small blood vessels in the kidneys and weakening their filtration function. This may lead to long-term kidney problems and potential kidney failure.

- **Weight Gain**

Unsurprisingly, consuming too much sugar causes an increase in insulin and glucose levels, leading to the storage of excess fat in the body.

- **Erectile Dysfunction**

Increased weight due to excessive sugar intake can lead to a drop in testosterone production, potentially causing erectile dysfunction.

- **Insulin Resistance**

Hidden sugars can disrupt the body's insulin resistance system, which regulates blood sugar levels. This disruption may increase the risk of developing diabetes.

Sugar Disguises in Processed Foods

Processed foods have become a prominent feature of modern lifestyle, offering convenience and a myriad of flavours. However, behind the enticing packaging lies a hidden danger – sugar. From frozen meals and canned soups to snacks and condiments, processed foods can be riddled with added sugars, preservatives, and artificial sweeteners. A good knowledge of food labels and nutritional information will help to decipher the hidden messages and enable more informed choices.

The World of Food Labels and Nutritional Information

Food labels are an excellent way to learn about the nutritional value of foods. They allow you to make good food choices. You can find good nutrition information on pre-packaged foods by looking at their labels, including:

- The nutrition facts table

- The list of ingredients

- The nutritional claims

1. **Nutrition Facts Table**

    The nutrition facts table is required to appear on most packaged food products. It helps you make informed food choices by comparing two similar products easily, finding out how many nutrients and calories a food contains, identifying foods with a little or a lot of a nutrient, and choosing foods suitable for special diets, such as diabetes diet.

The nutrition facts table provides information about the food for a given serving, usually the amount consumed in a single meal or snack. It indicates, in particular, the number of calories that a serving contains as well as the number of its main nutrients expressed in grams (g), milligrams (mg), micrograms (µg), or percentage of the daily value.

2. List of Ingredients

The ingredient list is on most pre-packaged products containing more than one ingredient. It lists all the ingredients in a packaged food in descending order of weight.

Studying the list of ingredients on a particular food item, especially the likes from a supermarket, enables you to know the exact amount of sugar a particular food contains. Since this list is in descending order of weight, it's easy to evaluate the amount of sugar in it and deduce whether it's healthy for you.

3. Nutritional Claims

A nutrition claim refers to the message that appears on food packaging. Manufacturers generally use two types of messages or claims:

- **Nutrient Content Claims**

These claims describe a food's nutritional value or benefit. For example, the statement 'Good source of iron' written on a product's packaging indicates that the food item will replenish you with the iron mineral, an essential micronutrient needed in your body.

- **Health Claims**

They describe the beneficial effects of a food or certain types of food on health. Here's an example of a health claim: 'This food is a good source of calcium. Adequate intake of calcium may reduce the risk of osteoporosis'.

Interestingly, food labels help you to discover disguised and hidden sugars in processed foods. Thus, do not hurriedly consume a pack of biscuits or a packaged cereal. Sit with the food label and go through the nutrition facts table, list of ingredients, as well as nutritional claims. This will help you tread with caution even as you indulge your cravings. However, By embracing whole foods and preparing meals from scratch, you can significantly reduce your sugar intake and nourish your body

The Emotional Connection

It's important to recognise that our relationship with sugar often extends beyond mere nutritional choices. Many of us turn to sugary treats for emotional comfort or reward. Understanding our emotional connection with sugar allows us to address the underlying reasons for our cravings.

Let's explore alternative ways to cope with stress, find solace, and celebrate without relying on sugar, which include but are not limited to the following:

1. Drink a glass of water.

2. Eat more protein.

3. Talk to a friend.

4. Avoid excess stress.

5. Identify and avoid your triggers.

6. Read a book or watch a comedy.

7. Take a bath and wrap yourself under a warm blanket.

8. Turn to a physical activity you enjoy, e.g., dancing, playing the guitar, etc.

By cultivating a mindful approach to your emotions and adopting healthier coping mechanisms, you can gradually reduce your reliance on sugar as a source of comfort.

As we conclude this chapter, I have uncovered the sweet saboteurs that lurk in our everyday lives. From the hidden sugars in our pantry to the deceptive beverages and processed foods, we have unmasked the culprits contributing to excessive sugar consumption. Armed with this newfound knowledge, you are more empowered to make conscious choices and prioritise your health and well-being.

In subsequent chapters, we will explore strategies to reduce sugar cravings, discover healthier alternatives, and establish sustainable habits leading to a balanced, sugar-smart lifestyle. It is essential to exercise moderation and discipline when it comes to sugar consumption, as it impacts various aspects of one's health. Resisting the allure of sugar can be challenging, but it is crucial to prioritise your well-being. Fortunately, there are healthy alternatives available to satisfy any sweet cravings you may have.

Chapter Three

CONQUERING SUGAR CRAVINGS

Having learnt about the detrimental effects of sugary diets, it is only wise that you also discover how to conquer your sugar cravings. In this chapter, we will explore effective strategies and practical tips to help you overcome the allure of sugary treats and establish healthier habits that support your well-being.

In today's world, sugar has become a predominant ingredient in our food, and it is almost effortless to slip into the trap of consuming excessive sugar. Consuming diets like beverages and hidden sugars in processed food will not produce positive results in the body. If allowed to persist, the impact of this seductive temptation will be detrimental to our health, hindering us from living a healthy and happy life.

The first step to fight against sugar cravings is understanding what excessive sugar intake does to your health. Afterwards, you set goals to take control of your sugar intake. While this will take effort, it is not impossible. You can take charge, make wise decisions, and foster an environment that supports healthy living. This is significant because the rewards of overcoming sugar cravings go far beyond a simple dietary shift; they pave the way to a fulfilling life. Keep in mind that moderate actions lead to massive transformations.

Strategies to Conquer Sugar Cravings

Understanding the origin of sugar cravings and how to conquer them is essential. Various factors, including physiological, psychological, and environmental triggers, can influence cravings. We will delve into the science behind cravings, exploring how our brains and bodies respond to sugar and the mechanisms that drive our desire for it. By gaining insight into our cravings, we can develop strategies to overcome them more effectively.

Since conquering sugar cravings is important, we must consider ways to achieve this goal. Some strategies we can employ are as follows:

1. **Understand Cravings**

   Have you ever wondered why resisting the allure of that slice of cake and a bowl of ice cream is so difficult? In the past, sweet-tasting meals were frequently a sign of a good energy source in nature, so our bodies have evolved to seek them out. This shows that our biology has a deep connection with sugar cravings. However, in the modern world, where sugar is cheap and widely accessible, this predisposition can become a problem.

While biological factors in sugar cravings are essential, emotional motivations are also worth considering. Many of us turn to sweets as a reward or solace in times of stress, boredom, or despair. This emotional attachment to sugar can become ingrained, resulting in a cycle of coping with stress by eating sugar.

Sugar addiction frequently results from a confluence of biological and mental elements. Eating sugar, especially in enormous amounts, causes an increase in our blood sugar levels followed by a drop in it. This crash causes hunger and sugar cravings, continuing the cycle of highs and lows.

Additionally, consuming sugary foods might constantly dull our taste buds, requiring us to take more significant doses of the sweet substance to produce the same delight. Sugar tolerance is the term for this occurrence. As the tolerance grows, the need for more sugar intensifies, which sets off a cycle in which an ever-increasing sugar intake is required to achieve the desired effect.

2. Mindful Eating

Practising mindful eating is a powerful tool for conquering sugar cravings. You can reconnect with your body and tune in to its nutritional needs by cultivating present-moment awareness during meals and snacks. Mindful eating involves savouring each bite, being attentive to hunger and fullness cues, and choosing foods that nourish and energise you. By focusing on the experience of eating, you can diminish impulsive cravings and make more conscious choices.

Mindful eating emanates from mindfulness, an old practice of many religions. Mindfulness involves intentionally focusing on your thoughts and emotions at the moment. In other words, mindful eating implies that your physical and emotional being is present for a better experience of your choice of food. Mindful eating also encourages you to make wise food choices that will help you conquer your cravings and choose foods that will satisfy and nourish your body.

By incorporating mindful eating into your daily life, you can change how you view food and gradually eliminate those nagging sugar cravings. However, mindful eating does not equate to a restricted diet. Rather, it implies that you can make deliberate decisions about your eating habits and nutrients by staying alert.

One core tenet of mindful eating is to approach your meals with an attitude free of bias. Instead of categorising foods as good or bad, observe your thoughts, feelings, and bodily sensations without judgement or value judgement.

Living a sugar-wise lifestyle involves making conscious choices about the foods you consume. Practising mindful eating is a vital component of this pursuit, a powerful tool to support you. By embracing mindful eating, you can cultivate a strong sense of being present during your meals and snacks, allowing you to reconnect with your body and tune in to its nutritional needs.

This is similar to having a trusted ally guiding you. As you savour each bite and pay close attention to your hunger and fullness cues, you become more aware and in control of your eating habits, making mindful and nourishing choices that align with your well-being. This mindful approach helps diminish impulsive sugar cravings, enabling you to navigate temptations and opt for healthier alternatives.

3. Balancing Macronutrients

Imbalances in your macronutrient intake, particularly the overconsumption of refined carbohydrates, can contribute to sugar cravings. Incorporating balanced protein, healthy fats, and complex carbohydrates into your meals and snacks is important. By doing so, you can stabilise your blood sugar levels, promote satiety, and reduce the likelihood of experiencing intense sugar cravings.

Understanding the role of macronutrients empowers you to create well-rounded, nourishing meals that support your overall health. Your body can suffer damage if your macronutrient intake is out of balance, especially if you consume excess refined carbohydrates. These quick jumps in blood sugar levels caused by these simple carbs in processed foods and sweet desserts result in energy dumps and subsequent sugar cravings. Breaking the pattern of this uncomfortable rollercoaster thus becomes difficult. The first step in reclaiming control over our nutritional choices is identifying the link between macronutrient imbalances and sugar cravings.

To prevent the effect of carbohydrate and sugar cravings, you need to incorporate a balanced mix of macronutrients in your meals. Let's discuss how each macronutrient contributes to curbing sugar cravings and supporting a healthy lifestyle.

- **Proteins**

It takes a longer time for proteins to digest in the body. However, incorporating sufficient proteins in your meals promotes satiety and helps stabilise blood sugar levels.

- **Healthy Fats**

There are misconceptions about the intake of fats in the body. Just as amounts of protein are important in a diet, healthy fats are also an important part of a balanced diet. They ensure you stay satisfied for extended periods. Healthy fats like avocados, nuts, seeds, olive oil, and fatty fish salmon can help prevent cravings triggered by hunger and enhance the flavour and texture of your meals.

- **Complex Carbohydrates**

Complex carbs provide a long and continuous release of energy instead of refined carbohydrates, which generate quick blood sugar increases. They offer a continual source of nutrition for our bodies because they are high in fibre, vitamins, and minerals. Excellent sources of complex carbs that can help regulate blood sugar levels and lessen sugar cravings include whole grains, vegetables, fruits, and legumes.

4. Healthy Alternatives

Discovering healthier alternatives to sugary treats is crucial in curbing cravings. Various options include fresh fruits, stevia or monk fruit, natural sweeteners, and healthy homemade snacks. Satisfying your sweet tooth with healthier alternatives provides a guilt-free indulgence while nourishing your body with vitamins, minerals, and fibre. Subsequently, we will discuss the importance of moderation, as even healthier sweet options should be consumed mindfully and in appropriate portions.

Here are some healthy food alternatives to consider adding to your diet:

- **Fresh Fruits**

Nature has blessed us with abundant sweet and delectable fruits that satisfy our desires while providing several health advantages. The selections range from luscious berries rich in antioxidants to crisp citrus fruits brimming with vitamin C. Various fresh fruits may appease your sweet cravings while offering a nourishing dose of critical nutrients, whether a juicy slice of watermelon on a warm summer day or a crisp apple delivering a pleasing crunch.

- **Various Natural Sweeteners**

Natural sweeteners like stevia or monk fruit can completely transform the situation for individuals looking for alternatives. These sweeteners, derived from plant sources, provide a delicious burst of sweetness without the negative consequences of consuming too much sugar.

Stevia, made from the leaves of the *Stevia rebaudiana*, has little effect on blood sugar levels while providing tremendous sweetness. The fruit of the *Siraitia grosvenorii* plant is used to make monk fruit extract, a natural, calorie-free sweetener for beverages and food. You can enjoy sweetness without sacrificing your health by embracing these natural sweeteners.

- **Homemade Snacks**

Making your snacks gives you control over the ingredients in what you eat. It also allows you to create healthy, nutrient-rich substitutes to satisfy your desires. Incorporating healthful ingredients like whole grains, nuts, seeds, and dried fruits allows you to create exquisite delights that satisfy your sweet tooth while being nutrient-dense. If you want a natural sweetness and energy boost, consider making your energy balls out of dates, almonds, and cacao. Also, you can bake oatmeal cookies with mashed bananas and cinnamon for a cosy and guilt-free treat.

While there are sweet and healthy food substitutes, it's important to also approach them mindfully and in moderation. Resist overeating by taking time with each bite and paying attention to your body cues that tell you when you are full. In other words, to keep a balanced approach to your eating choices, it is required that you keep practising moderation.

In this chapter, we have explored a range of strategies to conquer sugar cravings and develop a healthier relationship with food. By understanding the origins of cravings, practising mindful eating, balancing macronutrients, and discovering healthier alternatives, you lay the groundwork for sustainable change.

In the following chapters, we will delve deeper into the benefits of reducing sugar consumption, the importance of physical activity, and additional tools and techniques to further support your journey toward a sugar-wise lifestyle.

Chapter Four

REDUCING SUGAR CONSUMPTION – THE BASICS OF A BALANCED NUTRITION

There are numerous benefits to reducing your sugar consumption on your overall health, well-being, and quality of life. But first, let's see the steps you can take to reduce sugar consumption.

These steps have been proven to be effective in reducing sugar consumption. They have worked for me, and I believe they can also work for you. These practical steps include:

- **Eat Whole Foods**

  Gradually reduce and eliminate easy-to-make, least-effort-required meals from your diet because such foods are processed and high in sugar. Embrace a habit of cooking by yourself. Purchase fresh produce and whole foods that have not been processed, such as vegetables, poultry, fish, beans, lentils, brown rice, or plain yoghurts.

- ### **Replace Sugar in Your Recipes**

Perhaps you are preparing a nice homemade treat and following a recipe that advises you to add sugar to your preparation. Rather than follow the instructions, you can replace the sugar with healthy alternatives like mashed banana, honey, maple syrup, or even dates. These healthy foods are a good alternative because they taste naturally sweet.

- ### **Avoid Sugary Drinks**

I know! When the hawkers on the streets with bowls of assorted chilled drinks beckon to you, especially when you've been out all day and feel drained, please, by all means, try not to indulge that craving. When thirsty, hydrate yourself with water or unsweetened, low-fat milk instead of sugary drinks like sodas or syrups.

You can flavour your water by adding slices of citrus fruits such as lemon or orange or even fresh raspberries and mint leaves.

- ### **Choose Healthy Snacks**

Opt for healthy snacks if you feel hungry between lunch and dinner. Resist settling for cakes, biscuits, and all the readily available snacks with no nutritional value. Instead, eat healthy snacks such as nuts, low-fat cheese, plain yoghurt, or fresh fruit.

Benefits of Reducing Your Sugar Consumption

Let us uncover the positive impact of reducing sugar consumption. These benefits include increased energy and vitality, weight management and body composition, enhanced mental clarity and focus, improved dental health, and reduced risk of chronic diseases.

- **Increased Energy and Vitality**

  It is advisable to pay attention to the amount of sugar you ingest daily to stay healthy. According to figures from the World Health Organisation (WHO), the level of sugar consumed daily should not exceed 10% of the total energy intake per day. Yes! That energy drink is sweet and savoury in your mouth, but can you make an effort to stop taking it?

  Conversely, and I know this may surprise you, when you take less sugary drinks, you actually get more energy to perform your daily activities. Most energy promised by sugary drinks is fleeting and will do more harm than good. Excessive sugar consumption can lead to energy crashes and fluctuations in blood sugar levels.

  By reducing your sugar intake and opting for nutrient-dense foods, you can stabilise your energy levels and experience consistent vitality throughout the day. A balanced nutrition supports optimal energy levels and improves your overall well-being.

- **Weight Management and Body Composition**

  Sugar-rich diets are often associated with weight gain and increased body fat. Reducing your sugar intake can support healthy weight management and improve your body composition. In a later chapter, we will discuss the impact of sugar on your metabolism, the role of sugar in triggering over-eating, and how reducing sugar can contribute to maintaining a healthy weight.

Added sugars are digested at high speed and, thus, disrupt the work of your body, e.g., blood sugar fluctuates, hormones are not secreted as they should, and weight gain sometimes even increases to obesity. Excess sugar raises fat (triglycerides) levels in the blood, cholesterol levels, and blood pressure. This is called metabolic syndrome, a collection of factors that increase the risk of developing heart disease.

Consuming sugary foods and drinks activates your brain's reward system; it is this same system that can lead to addiction. How many people around you love cakes? Or candy? Or soft drinks? Why do people love sugary foods and drinks so much? Why don't most of us have the same love for, say, kola nut? The answer is in your brain.

When you eat something that contains sugar, the sugars activate the sweet taste receptors in your taste buds. These receptors send a signal to your brain, which processes the sensory information and understands that you are tasting something sweet. Alas! The pleasure tricks your brain into wanting more sugary food that makes you feel good, but unfortunately, it plunges you deeper into unhealthy living.

By disrupting the metabolism, excess sugar makes you fatter than necessary. It causes a secretion of insulin (whose role is to bring glucose into the cells to bring blood sugar to a normal value), which leads to a storage mechanism of sugar and fat storage. Reducing and stopping sugar, therefore, contributes to weight loss.

By reducing sugar, you will also reduce any addiction and the cravings that result from it; when you replace sugar with nutritious whole foods, your hormones naturally regulate, sending signals to the brain when you've had enough to eat. As a result, you'll lose weight effortlessly.

- **Enhanced Mental Clarity and Focus**

High sugar consumption has been linked to cognitive issues such as brain fog, poor concentration, and decreased mental clarity. By reducing your sugar intake and choosing foods that support brain health, you can enhance your mental clarity, focus, and cognitive function.

The role of sugar in brain health is paramount as it is a powerful stimulant for our brain. This is why a cascade of chemical messages is set in motion when you taste a spoonful of ice cream, chocolate bar, cake, and other sugary foods. These messages activate the famous reward circuit, located at the heart of the brain and composed of the ventral tegmental area (VTA) and the nucleus accumbens.

The activation of the reward circuit leads to the release of dopamine, a neurotransmitter that is the source of sensations of pleasure. This circuit pushes you to reproduce activities essential to your survival, such as eating, sleeping, and making love. In the case of sugar, the connections between the nucleus accumbens and the cortex generate a decision to continue taking sugar.

There are quite a few dietary strategies you can adopt to promote optimal mental well-being. One surefire way is to adopt a healthy, varied, balanced diet with adequate fruits and vegetables. Other ways include keeping regular schedules and taking the time to eat calmly, avoiding drinks containing sugar, caffeine, or alcohol; do so in moderation if you consume them. Adequate nutrition provides the necessary nutrients that help bring energy and vitality to the body, thus promoting good mental health.

- **Improved dental health**

There is a close-knit relationship between sugar consumption and tooth decay. When you consume excessive amounts of sugar, the sugar molecules interact with saliva, providing a breeding ground for bacteria in the mouth. This can result in the formation of plaque on the teeth, which, if left untreated, can advance into cavities.

By consistently brushing your teeth, you can decrease the likelihood of this occurrence and reduce the risk of developing gum disease over time. Excessive sugar consumption contributes to tooth decay and cavities; reducing sugar intake helps protect your teeth and promotes better oral health.

- **Reduced Risk of Chronic Diseases**

High sugar intake has been associated with an increased risk of developing chronic conditions such as type 2 diabetes, heart disease, and certain cancers. Research has proven that individuals with at least 25% sugar in their calorie intake are twice as likely to die from cardiovascular disease compared to those with only 10%.

Now, that's shocking when almost everything we eat contains some added sugar, which is a significant factor in causing high blood pressure as it increases the work rate of the heart and arteries and can cause long-term damage over time. Ingesting food or beverages that contain excessive added sugars places additional strain on the heart, which can be potentially life-threatening for individuals with an unhealthy diet.

Enhancing your dietary choices by obtaining sugar from fruits rather than saturated fatty foods will diminish the risk of experiencing a heart attack. However, lowering sugar consumption can help mitigate these health risks and enable you to lead a healthier lifestyle.

Lastly, research suggests excessive sugar consumption may also contribute to mood swings, anxiety, and depression. Sugary foods are often high in calories but low in essential nutrients. Moderating your sugar intake allows you to focus on a more balanced diet, incorporating nutrient-rich foods that support your overall health to experience improved mental well-being and mood stability.

Note moderation is key. It is important to be mindful of hidden sugars in processed foods and beverages and to opt for natural, whole foods whenever possible. Furthermore, consulting with a healthcare professional or registered dietitian can provide personalised guidance on maintaining a healthy diet.

Chapter Five

THE ROLE OF PHYSICAL ACTIVITY

In this chapter, we shift our focus to the role of physical activity in a sugar-wise lifestyle. Living a sugar-wise lifestyle involves making conscious choices to reduce sugar consumption and prioritise overall health and well-being. While dietary changes are crucial, you should also consider the role of physical activity. Physical activity is a powerful tool for long-term sugar reduction and overall well-being.

The role of exercise in blood sugar regulation, weight management, mood enhancement, energy levels, habit formation, and social engagement is essential for an active lifestyle. Even small steps can yield significant benefits, so start today and make physical activity an integral part of your sugar-wise journey.

The Role of Physical Activity in an Active Lifestyle

While reducing sugar consumption is crucial for your health, combining it with regular exercise amplifies the benefits. We explore how physical activity supports overall well-being and aids in maintaining a balanced and healthy lifestyle.

1. Exercise and Sugar Regulation

Regular exercise regulates blood sugar levels and promotes overall metabolic health. It also plays a significant role in regulating blood sugar levels by facilitating glucose uptake by muscles. Exercise enhances insulin sensitivity and allows our bodies to manage sugar in the bloodstream more effectively.

Here are the impacts of exercise in promoting the regulation of blood sugar levels.

- **Insulin Sensitivity**

Insulin is a hormone responsible for regulating blood sugar levels by facilitating glucose uptake into cells. Physical activity enhances insulin sensitivity, making the body more responsive to insulin's actions. Regular exercise helps the body use insulin more effectively, improving blood sugar control and reducing insulin resistance.

- ## Sugar Regulation

Exercises like aerobic or cardiovascular exercise can help to increase the heart rate and breathing because it involves continuous movement. This type of exercise has many benefits for sugar regulation. Muscles require additional energy during aerobic exercise, prompting the body to utilise glucose as fuel. This process helps lower blood sugar levels and increases insulin sensitivity.

In addition, brisk walking, running, cycling, swimming, or dancing for at least 150 minutes per week is recommended to promote sugar regulation.

- ## Resistance Training and Sugar Regulation

Resistance training, strength or weight training, involves working against resistance to build and strengthen muscles. While this may not directly impact blood sugar levels during exercise, resistance training offers long-term benefits for sugar regulation. It helps increase muscle mass, improving glucose uptake and muscle storage. Over time, this can lead to enhanced insulin sensitivity and better blood sugar control.

I recommend you include resistance training exercises, such as weightlifting, body weight exercises, or using resistance bands, two to three times per week to support sugar regulation.

- **High-Intensity Interval Training (HIIT) and Sugar Regulation**

High-Intensity Interval Training (HIIT) involves alternating between short bursts of intense exercise and brief recovery periods. HIIT has gained popularity because of its effectiveness in improving cardiovascular fitness and metabolic health. Studies have shown that HIIT can enhance sugar regulation by improving insulin sensitivity and increasing muscle glucose uptake. Incorporating HIIT workouts, such as sprint intervals, circuit training, or Tabata training, into your exercise routine can be a time-efficient and beneficial strategy for sugar control.

- **Timing and Consistency**

Consistency is vital when it comes to exercise and sugar regulation. Regular physical activity helps maintain steady blood sugar levels and improves overall metabolic health. Aim for a balanced exercise routine that includes aerobic exercise, resistance training, and HIIT workouts. Additionally, spacing out exercise sessions throughout the week and incorporating physical activity into daily routines can support stable blood sugar control.

2. Weight Management and Body Composition

Reduced sugar consumption and regular physical activity, such as cardiovascular exercise and strength training, support weight management and improve body composition. Exercise increases calorie expenditure, builds lean muscle mass, and promotes a healthy metabolic rate. Incorporating exercise into our routine can enhance our body's ability to maintain a healthy weight, reduce the risk of developing conditions like insulin resistance, obesity, and type 2 diabetes, and optimise overall health.

Adopting a programme of regular physical activity is crucial for promoting a healthier lifestyle in terms of weight control and body composition. This includes reducing sugar intake while exercising your heart and muscles and strengthening your body. Combining these techniques has a synergistic effect that helps with weight loss and changes the makeup of our bodies for the better.

Let's clarify how exercise contributes to these outcomes by delving into the mechanics of this phenomenon. First, exercise causes a rise in caloric expenditure. When you exercise, your body burns more calories than it would if you remained sedentary. This calorie-burning mechanism is crucial to weight control because, when combined with a balanced diet, it helps create a caloric deficit that, in turn, promotes weight loss and prevents weight gain.

Exercise is also a crucial advocate for fostering a healthy metabolic rate. A higher metabolic rate suggests that your body can use nutrients, including sugars and fats, more effectively. The ability of your body to properly handle these nutrients enhances a healthy metabolic rate, which lowers the likelihood that extra fat and sugar will be stored in addition to the possibility of illnesses like insulin resistance, obesity, and type 2 diabetes.

Making regular exercise a part of your lifestyle puts you on the path to improving your overall health. In addition to helping with weight control and improving body composition, it has a wide range of additional health advantages. Exercise is a comprehensive strategy for living a happier and more satisfying life since it positively impacts overall health beyond physical well-being.

3. Mood and Stress Management

Physical activity is known to have positive effects on mood and stress management. Regular exercise releases endorphins, the 'feel-good' hormones, which can ease stress, anxiety, and symptoms of depression. Here, we will discuss the impact of exercise on mental well-being and its role in supporting a balanced emotional state.

One of the primary ways exercise promotes mental health is by releasing endorphins. Endorphins are neurotransmitters that act as natural mood lifters and pain relievers. When you engage in physical activity, especially aerobic exercises like running, swimming, or cycling, your body releases these feel-good chemicals, creating a sense of euphoria and easing stress and anxiety. This is often called the runner's high – heightened happiness and relaxation experienced during or after vigorous exercise.

Exercise serves as a powerful stress reducer. In today's fast-paced and demanding world, stress has become prevalent, taking a toll on mental health. Engaging in physical activity helps combat the negative effects of stress by promoting the release of tension and pent-up energy, allowing the mind to relax and refocus. Regular exercise also helps regulate cortisol levels, the hormone associated with stress, further promoting a calmer and more balanced emotional state.

4. Improve Insulin Sensitivity

Insulin sensitivity refers to how sensitive the cells are to the hormone insulin's effects. However, regular physical activities improve insulin sensitivity, enabling cells to efficiently utilise glucose from the bloodstream. It prevents insulin resistance, often associated with excessive sugar consumption.

When you eat, especially foods high in carbohydrates, your blood sugar levels rise, prompting the pancreas to release insulin. Insulin then acts as a key that unlocks your cells, allowing glucose to penetrate and be converted to energy.

In individuals with high insulin sensitivity, their cells respond efficiently to insulin, meaning that only a tiny amount of insulin is required to facilitate glucose uptake from the bloodstream into the cells. It benefits overall health because it helps maintain stable blood sugar levels and reduces the risk of developing insulin-related health issues. Here are five popular ways to improve your insulin sensitivity:

- **Regular Exercise**

Engaging in both aerobic exercises (e.g., walking, running, cycling) and strength training has been shown to increase insulin sensitivity. Physical activity helps muscles better utilise glucose for energy, reducing the need for higher insulin levels.

- **Get Enough Sleep**

Poor sleep patterns and inadequate sleep are associated with insulin resistance. Strive for 7-9 hours of quality sleep per night.

- **Manage Stress**

Chronic stress can contribute to insulin resistance—practice stress-reduction techniques such as meditation, yoga, deep breathing exercises, or spending time in nature.

- **Eat a Balanced Diet**

Focus on consuming whole, nutrient-dense foods low in refined carbohydrates and added sugars. Emphasise fibre-rich foods like vegetables, fruits, whole grains, and legumes, which can help slow down glucose absorption and stabilise blood sugar levels.

- **Maintain a Healthy Weight**

Excess body weight, especially abdominal fat, is closely linked to insulin resistance. You can significantly improve insulin sensitivity by achieving and maintaining a healthy weight through a balanced diet and exercise.

- **Overall Well-Being**

Physical activities contribute to overall well-being by boosting mood, improving cognitive function, and reducing the risk of chronic disease. When your overall well-being is satisfied through exercise, you may be less inclined to rely on sugary foods for emotional comfort or stress relief.

Achieving a high level of overall well-being is a dynamic and ongoing process involving balance, fulfilment, and a sense of purpose.

Key Dimensions That Contribute to Overall Well-Being

- **Physical Well-Being**

This dimension involves preventive healthcare and caring for one's physical health, including proper nutrition, regular exercise, and adequate sleep. Maintaining a healthy body helps enhance energy levels, reduce the risk of chronic diseases, and promote longevity.

- **Mental Well-Being**

Mental well-being is about having a positive and stable mental state. It includes emotional resilience, coping with stress, and maintaining mental clarity and focus. Engaging in activities stimulating the mind, such as learning new skills or hobbies, can also contribute to mental well-being.

- **Emotional Well-Being**

Emotional well-being involves understanding and managing one's emotions healthily and constructively. It is about experiencing a range of emotions while being able to express them appropriately and seeking support when needed.

- **Social Well-Being**

Social well-being is the quality of an individual's relationships and connection with others. Positive social interactions, meaningful friendships, and a sense of belonging to a community all contribute to social well-being.

- **Environmental Well-Being**

Environmental well-being involves living in a safe, clean, and supportive environment. Being connected to nature and caring for the environment can also influence overall well-being.

Improving your overall well-being requires conscious efforts and ongoing self-assessment in these different dimensions. Taking small steps to address each aspect can have a cumulative and positive impact on one's quality of life. A well-balanced approach to life, with attention to physical, mental, emotional, social, and environmental needs, contributes to higher overall well-being and a more fulfilling and satisfying life.

CONQUERING CRAVINGS AND MAKING MINDFUL CHOICES

Cravings can be a formidable challenge on your journey towards a sugar-wise lifestyle. However, they also serve as important messages your body sends to help maintain inner balance. When you feel a craving, do not consider it a weakness; rather, question what your body wants and why. It is also crucial not to give in to temptations.

By understanding your cravings and developing a mindful approach, you can gain control over your choices and stay on track toward a healthier, balanced life.

Unravelling the Craving Puzzle

Cravings often arise from biological, psychological, and environmental factors. These factors are known as primary food. Primary food refers to personal, emotional, physical, and spiritual non-food satisfaction you need to feel happy, secure, and fulfilled.

Often, most people indulge in their cravings to fill the primary food void. Being unhappy in a relationship, being bored with their jobs, participating in an exercise routine that is not enough for their bodies, or a lack of sleep due to anxiety can all cause constant specific cravings.

Let's delve into the various triggers that can lead to cravings. Triggers like stress, emotions, habit, and sensory cues are mental triggers that influence your brain's decisions at the unconscious level.

- **Stress**

  The stress hormone, known as cortisol, is a potential trigger of cravings. When you have high cortisol levels, it's natural to crave sweet or carb-heavy foods. You can reduce stress by getting adequate sleep, taking frequent breaks, exercising moderately, and listening to soothing music, thereby reducing cravings.

- **Emotions**

  Evidence suggests that highly palatable foods, especially those high in fat and sugar, can cause a reaction in the brain similar to that caused by opioids. Yes, a delicious slice of chocolate cake can feel as good as drugs, and that's why many resort to taking chocolate when stressed, all because of this 'high' feeling it gives them. They tend to call many of these foods comfort food, but that definition can be a bit nebulous.

The choice of food is deeply personal. Foods that comfort will depend on a person's cultural background, taste preferences, and personal experiences. We also know that foods can induce nostalgia that transports us back to simpler, better times.

So it's not surprising that during an uncertain time when many are desperate for some relief and comfort, they turn to their cravings. And this is how they allow emotions to dictate their cravings, knowingly or unknowingly.

- **Habit**

Every time you escape difficult situations by relying on food cravings, you gradually build an unhealthy eating habit. Bad habits can be the bane of one's existence, especially if one cannot unlearn that habit. Habits are difficult to break, so you should stop using food cravings (sugar, in this case) to break out of challenging situations. Your body gets used to it in no time, and every time you're stressed or your emotions get the better of you, your brain tricks your palates into seeking sugary foods.

- **Sensory Cues**

Additives and preservatives are proven to affect a part of the brain known as the appestat that controls the feeling of hunger. Processed ingredients can trick the appetite into telling you to eat more. That is why some people consume more fast food than reasonable.

Cravings are an indication that something is out of balance in your life. Therefore, always aim to balance your life, blood sugar levels, fluid intake, and exercise, as this should help eliminate cravings. By understanding the root causes of your cravings, you can gain insights that enable you to address them effectively.

Mindfulness and Craving Awareness

Mindfulness plays a pivotal role in conquering cravings. Mindful eating is a great way to curb cravings. As discussed in Chapter Three, mindful eating involves paying attention to your thoughts, emotions, and bodily sensations as you consume food. By cultivating awareness and being fully present, you can better discern the true nature of your cravings, recognise their fleeting nature, and make conscious choices that align with your health goals.

Strategies for Managing Cravings

Managing cravings requires a combination of proactive and reactive strategies. There are several basic strategies to employ when managing your cravings. The first involves tracking your daily habits. For example, is there a specific time of day when you feel particularly hungry? Do you feel like eating sweets at night? Do you immediately turn to food as a coping mechanism when faced with a stressful situation? Be as objective as possible when answering these and similar questions.

After tracking your cravings, the next step is eliminating unhealthy substances from your diet. For example, you could turn to a bowl of fresh fruit as an alternative to a chocolate bar or soda. It is also advisable to include a lot of fibre in your diet. The fibre will give you a feeling of fullness for an extended period. Finally, remember to drink plenty of water. This keeps you hydrated, and the water helps relieve hunger and unnecessary cravings.

Additionally, there are mindfulness-based techniques that you can use to address your cravings. These techniques include deep breathing, practising self-compassion, and redirecting your attention to healthier alternatives.

- **Deep Breathing**

  By engaging in slow, deliberate breaths, you can significantly reduce the intensity of your cravings. Counting your breaths or adopting a rhythmic breathing pattern like the 4-7-8 method can divert your focus from the craving, easing your agitation and promoting relaxation.

  Moreover, the 4-7-8 technique offers added benefits. As you breathe out longer than you breathe in, your heart rate slows, ushering in a profound sense of calm. So, next time a craving strikes, take charge with deep breathing. Consider it your ally in the fight against cravings and stress.

- **Practise Self-Compassion**

  In leading a sugar-smart lifestyle, know you are not alone. To encourage yourself and exceed your set milestones, practise self-talk and self-compassion. Stay mindful of your nutrition, weight, and health objectives. Remember, a food craving is merely a thought - the power to respond lies entirely in your hands.

- ### Redirect to Healthier Alternatives

  If you yearn for a food you can't control in small portions, opt for a wholesome and delightful substitute. For instance, if you crave the satisfying crunch of potato chips, consider snacking on carrots or even crispy fried plantains. To quench your thirst and curb cravings, go for bariatric-friendly beverages like water, herbal tea, or decaffeinated low-calorie drinks – they will keep you hydrated and assist in managing cravings.

Building a Supportive Environment

Creating a supportive environment can significantly impact your ability to conquer cravings and make mindful choices. Here, we will examine the influence of your surroundings, including the availability of sugary foods, social influences, and the power of social support.

- ### The Influence of Your Surroundings

  You often indulge in habits you once eschewed, all because you're still in the same environment where you built those habits. You must create or seek a supportive environment to conquer your sugar cravings.

  For instance, if you live in a house where sugar is always available in the pantry, try to stay clear of the pantry or take the things you'll personally need to your room. The availability of sugary foods can hinder your ability to overcome your cravings.

- **The Power of Social Support**

  Having a like-minded community on the same journey as you helps achieve faster results. Let the supportive people in your life know you're tackling unhealthy cravings. It will enable them to support you more and with intentional efforts to help you manage your cravings better.

  By surrounding yourself with individuals who share your commitment to a sugar-smart lifestyle and creating an environment that promotes healthier choices, you set yourself up for success.

As we conclude this chapter, you must understand that conquering cravings and making mindful choices are essential to your sugar-wise journey. By unravelling the complexities of cravings, cultivating mindfulness, implementing strategies to manage them, and building a supportive environment, you can regain control over your choices and forge a path toward lasting change.

Remember, conquering cravings is not about complete elimination or strict deprivation. It is about developing a healthy relationship with food, understanding your triggers, and making empowered choices that support your overall well-being. With mindfulness as your guide, you can navigate the temptations and challenges that come your way, staying true to your commitment to a sugar-wise lifestyle. As you progress on your healthy journey, embrace the power to conquer cravings and make mindful choices that nourish your body and soul.

Cheers to a future of intentional cravings, conscious choices, and balanced and healthy living.

Chapter Seven

NURTURING A SUSTAINABLE SUGAR-WISE LIFESTYLE

So far, we have explored the impact of sugar on health, strategies to conquer cravings, the role of physical activity, and practical tools for a sugar-wise lifestyle. It's time to focus on nurturing a sustainable approach to long-term success. We will also delve into the importance of having the right mindset, self-compassion, and support systems to cultivate a sustainable sugar-wise lifestyle.

Living a sugar-wise lifestyle refers to adopting a way of life that is mindful and responsible regarding sugar consumption while promoting sustainability. It involves making conscious choices and developing habits that prioritise personal health and contribute to the well-being of the environment and society. In this chapter, we'll discuss some critical aspects of nurturing a sustainable sWugar-wise lifestyle.

Shifting Mindset and Beliefs

Your mindset and beliefs are pivotal to your ability to adopt and sustain a sugar-smart lifestyle. The power of positive thinking, self-belief, and reframing your relationship encourages a sugar-smart lifestyle. By shifting your mindset from restriction to abundance and focusing on the benefits of reducing sugar intake, you can cultivate a sustainable approach rooted in self-care and well-being for an extended period. Here are some steps to take to achieve your desired result.

- **Educate Yourself**

  Start by learning about the harmful effects of high sugar intake on your health and environment. Understanding how sugar impacts your health motivates you to make positive changes.

- **Set Clear Goals**

  Define your aim for adopting a sustainable sugar-wise lifestyle. Set smart and realistic goals to gradually reduce sugar intake and make more sustainable choices.

- **Read Labels**

  Pay close attention to the labels on food and beverage products. Look for hidden sugars and opt for items with low sugar content. This will help you make better choices and reduce your sugar consumption.

- **Prepare Your Meals**

  This gives you control over the ingredients in your meal and the quantity you use. Also, instead of refined sugar, you can opt for honey, maple syrup, and stevia.

- **Celebrate Your Wins**

  Be kind to yourself while you go through this transition. Celebrate your achievements no matter how small, and don't get discouraged by occasional slip-ups. Shifting your mindset and beliefs will take time and effort; hence, you should be patient.

Gradual Reduction

Learning and educating yourself about the hidden sugar in your diet and understanding its impact on consuming excess sugar will lead you to a gradual reduction of your sugar intake. The knowledge will empower you to make informed decisions about your sugar intake rather than trying to eliminate it all at once. This allows your taste buds to adjust and makes your transition more sustainable.

In reducing your sugar intake, critically examine your diet to understand the quantity of added sugar you consume. Read labels because there is hidden sugar in so many processed foods. This is essential to your journey in living a sustainable sugar-wise lifestyle.

While on the path to living a healthy life, eating based on your emotions will hinder your progress toward a reduced sugar intake. However, you are good to go if you can learn alternative ways to manage stress. When left unaddressed, emotional eating will lead to increased sugar consumption. Some tips that can help you cope with stress rather than consuming excessive sugar are exercises, meditation, or spending time with loved ones.

Furthermore, you need friends, family, or online communities on your journey to reduce sugar consumption. Seeking support from specific people will help you stay motivated and accountable. Remember, gradual changes are more sustainable in the long run. Take it one step at a time. It's okay to have occasional indulgences. The bottom line is making healthier choices most of the time and staying mindful of your sugar intake. And at the end of the day, it becomes part of your sustained sugar-wise lifestyle.

Practising Self-Compassion

As discussed in the previous chapter, you need self-compassion. Embarking on any lifestyle change requires self-compassion and forgiveness. You'll learn about the importance of being gentle with yourself while on the journey toward a sugar-wise lifestyle. It's essential to acknowledge that setbacks may occur. Practising self-compassion allows you to learn without judgement or self-criticism. By fostering a supportive and kind inner dialogue, you can overcome obstacles and maintain motivation in the face of challenges.

Practising self-compassion helps you to develop a positive attitude towards your progress. When your sugar consumption goals are not going as planned, forgive yourself and accept the situation. Don't criticise and judge yourself; learn from your shortcomings and move on.

Note that cultivating a positive attitude and self-compassion can foster your relationship with food while on the journey to living a sustainable lifestyle.

Dr Kristin Neff, who introduced the concept of self-compassion, discovered that self-compassion solves negative self-talk and is a helpful tool for reducing depression, stress, and anxiety. Hence, you should embrace it on your healthy living journey.

Here are a few more reasons to be gentle with yourself as you move through the path of reducing your sugar intake.

- **Sustainable Progress**

  Making significant changes to your routine and body takes time and consistent effort. However, being gentle with yourself means recognising that progress might not always be linear, and there may be setbacks. Extending grace to yourself will help you bounce back from slip-ups as you continue sustainably working towards your goals.

- **Positive Mindset**

  Being gentle with yourself fosters a positive mindset essential for long-term success—disallow negative self-talk, which only leads to guilt and shame. Overcoming self-criticism creates a more supportive and fulfilling environment, increasing your chances of success.

- **Stress Reduction**

  Being gentle with yourself helps to reduce stress and promote a healthier relationship with food, which is crucial for making rational and balanced food choices.

- **Better Decision-Making**

When you are gentle with yourself, you make better decisions based on what's best for your well-being rather than out of pressure.

- **Improved Mental and Physical Health**

Gentle self-care practices and being mindful of sugar consumption can positively affect your mental and physical well-being. Living a sugar-wise lifestyle is about creating sustainable habits and making choices that promote health and balance. Thus, you should be patient, celebrate your successes, and be kind to yourself when facing challenges. Every small step towards a healthier relationship with sugar is a step in the right direction.

Building a Supportive Network

Surrounding yourself with a supportive network can significantly enhance your chances of success. The importance of seeking support from friends, family, or online communities who share similar goals in building a supportive network must be emphasised. Having individuals who understand your journey, offer encouragement, and provide accountability can significantly impact your ability to sustain a sugar-wise lifestyle. In other words, finding accountability partners to support one another's journey is vital.

Here are some reasons why having a strong support system is essential in nurturing your sugar-wise lifestyle.

- Being surrounded by like-minded individuals who share the same commitment, goals, and objectives is essential. Together, you form a powerful force and reinforce each other's choices, encouraging perseverance, especially in difficult times.

- There is abundant shared knowledge and experiences when you have the right supportive network. Members of your community share practical tips, coping strategies, and tested recipes that have worked for them.

- A supportive network offers continuous motivation. When low on determination, your peers can uplift you with inspiring stories and encouraging words.

- Healthy competition can arise within a network. It is not the competition where you envy others because you think they are doing better. This kind is one where observing the achievements of others makes you eager to meet your goals.

- Finally, every achievement, no matter how small, deserves to be celebrated. Whether it's resisting an alluring treat at a party or staying sugar-free all month, these milestones are applauded and rewarded by the entire community.

Celebrating Progress and Milestones

Recognising and celebrating your progress and milestones is crucial for maintaining motivation and sustaining long-term change. The significance of celebrating every success cannot be exaggerated. By acknowledging your achievements and rewarding yourself in non-food-related ways, you reinforce positive behaviour and maintain enthusiasm for your sugar-wise journey.

Celebrating your wins, no matter how small, is a wise practice. This simple act boosts your confidence and motivates you to do more. One way to celebrate progress and milestones on your journey to nurturing a sustainable sugar-wise lifestyle is by hosting friends and families to celebrate your achievements. Remember to also share your journey with them.

Another way is to set up a reward system. Treat yourself to something you enjoy most for reaching your sugar-wise goals. It could be taking yourself out on a spa treatment, taking a photo shoot, or visiting a bookstore. Also, remember to plan and prepare your meals beforehand to have more control over the ingredients. Avoid relying on processed sugary options. This is a key factor in cultivating a sustainable sugar-wise lifestyle.

In all, be patient with yourself and celebrate small victories along the way. With commitment and perseverance, you can develop healthy habits beneficial to your overall health and well-being.

Chapter Eight

NAVIGATING SOCIAL SITUATIONS AND CHALLENGES

In this chapter, we will address the social dynamics and challenges that can arise when trying to lead a sugar-smart lifestyle. We will explore strategies for navigating social situations, dealing with peer pressure, and overcoming common hurdles to ensure that your sugar-smart choices align with your overall well-being.

Strategies for Navigating Social Situations

As humans, we are social beings and cannot do without meeting others occasionally; thus, maintaining discipline may be difficult if you are on a solo journey to leading a healthier lifestyle.

Communicating your intentions and goals effectively to friends, family, and colleagues is crucial in navigating social situations. Hence, it is important to have open and honest communication with others about your lifestyle choices, assert boundaries, and educate others about the benefits of a sugar-smart lifestyle. By effectively communicating your needs, you can garner support and understanding from those around you.

- **Open and honest communication**

  Communication has to be a two-way street for it to be deemed successful. If you're trying to cut back on your sugar consumption, it is important to let the people you interact with the most know about your lifestyle change. That way, they are able to understand your reactions to certain happenings and know better not to get offended by them. By understanding your motives, they encourage you to do more and aim toward your goals.

- **Asserting your boundaries**

  Setting boundaries is another important aspect of navigating social situations. Boundaries keep you unwavering and attuned to your goals. By setting boundaries, you let people know to what extent they can interfere with your personal choices. If you want to go on an indefinite sugar strike, you must set boundaries even within your family. This is so that when your meal is being prepared, they know your servings must come without any traces of sugar. That's a typical example of setting boundaries within the context of developing a sugar-smart lifestyle.

- **Educating others about leading a sugar-smart lifestyle**

One thing is to start this intentional journey of leading a sugar-smart lifestyle on your own; another is to educate others about the importance of joining the train. By and by, anyone taking charge of their eating habits and purposefully reducing their sugar intake is on the way to living a healthier and stronger life. So, propagating the gospel helps free more people from the shackles of excessive sugar consumption while navigating social situations seamlessly and winning at your goals of leading a sugar-smart lifestyle.

Making Smart Choices in Social Settings

Social gatherings and events often present challenges when making sugar-smart choices. In this section, we will explore strategies for making healthier selections at parties, restaurants, and other social settings. Scanning menus beforehand and being mindful of portion sizes and alternative options can help you confidently navigate social situations and stay true to your sugar-smart goals.

Here are other tips for a healthier eating approach when outdoors:

- Prioritise eating before heading out: Make sure to consume healthy foods at home to avoid indulging in sugar-filled meals at an event you attend.

- Set limits on your food and drink intake: Consider adopting a two-plate and a two-drink limit to maintain moderation during your outing.

- Plan your meal: If possible, check the menu in advance and make wise, healthy choices before arriving at the venue.

- Stay hydrated, and include fruits and vegetables in your diet: Fruits and veggies are low in calories, making them an excellent choice for the sugar-smart individual. Consider adding them to your diet. Also, don't forget to drink enough water.

- Begin with a substantial salad before your main course: You can opt for lighter dressings to keep the calorie count in check while enjoying rich flavours.

- Keep a food log to increase your awareness of what you consume.

- Avoid alcohol, as it only comes with empty calories. Remember, you can still have a great time without alcohol intake.

- If you are attending a potluck-style party, prepare something healthy and bring it with you.

Dealing With Peer Pressure

Peer pressure can sometimes pose obstacles to your sugar-smart journey. In this section, we will discuss techniques for handling peer pressure to stay committed to your goals. By maintaining assertiveness, suggesting alternative activities, or bringing healthier options to gatherings, you can withstand external pressures and stay on track with your sugar-smart lifestyle.

When you find yourself surrounded by people consuming specific foods or excessively drinking alcohol, you may be tempted to join them. The reason behind this is quite clear—being part of the group is enjoyable. A sense of comfort and belonging always emerges from being with a group. However, conforming to the crowd's behaviour can lead to harmful decisions that can negatively impact your health. Moreover, when others actively encourage you to participate, staying committed to your own priorities becomes even more challenging.

Here are a few helpful tips on dealing with peer pressure to stay committed to your goal of leading a sugar-smart lifestyle:

1. **Take time to contemplate what holds significance in your life**

   Allocate fifteen minutes to ponder and respond to the following prompts. I recommend writing down your answers:

   - What destination do you aspire to reach in your health and wellness journey?

   - Are there people around you who have hindered your progress toward your goals? If so, in what ways have they made an impact on you?

   - What aspects do you value in your relationship with these people? Additionally, identify any specific roles you may hold in that relationship.

   This activity becomes particularly valuable when preparing for circumstances where you anticipate encountering additional peer pressure, such as during a vacation with friends and family or throughout the holiday season.

2. Practise portion control during challenging situations

Imagine that you have successfully maintained a sugar-smart routine in your diet. Your birthday comes around, and your co-workers surprise you with a cake. I believe you will feel thankful and compelled to indulge in a piece—it's your special day, after all! However, an inner voice may remind you of your journey to leading a sugar-smart lifestyle and your progress so far. It may urge you not to jeopardise it.

To take control of the situation, you can opt for only a small piece of the cake. You can suggest cutting that piece yourself or politely request a half-sized portion. If you are served a larger piece, don't hesitate to take only a small portion. Remember, even a smaller serving of dessert can satisfy you, allowing you to maintain the hard work you have invested in your health journey.

Overcoming Setbacks and Staying Motivated

Setbacks are a normal part of any lifestyle change. Here, we will discuss strategies for overcoming setbacks, staying motivated, and getting back on track after slip-ups. We will explore the importance of resilience, learning from setbacks, and reframing them as opportunities for growth.

When setbacks shift your firm footing, it is natural to want to throw in the towel and just give up. However, if you do so, how will you reach the end of your goal? How will you see that journey to the end and be able to recount the experience to someone else? That would be impossible. Hence, it is important to maintain the course and get back on track even after slipping up. Remember that failure is not when you go off course but when you refuse to get back up after failing.

To overcome setbacks, you need to be resilient. Resilience is the ability to stay strong in the face of adversity. When you are resilient, you doggedly pursue your goals and dance on the waves rather than allow them to sweep you away.

On your sugar-smart journey, you need to remain resilient because, as I established in previous chapters, you cannot totally avoid sugar. More often than not, it will still find its way through, primarily through packaged foods and other hidden sugar sources. Hence, resilience to stay focused and not waver has to be one of your coping mechanisms on this journey.

It is not enough to overcome setbacks. You have to also learn from them and reframe them as opportunities for growth. In reality, setbacks are an inescapable adventure we all go through at one point or another in our personal or professional lives. So, how can you deal with such limitations? First, you have to acknowledge that a setback exists.

For instance, if you've gone back to consuming sugar excessively, pause and consider how long you harboured that setback. This motivates you to escape from it as fast as you can and know what level of damage the setback has wreaked and how best to combat it.

Next, use the setback as an opportunity to gain new knowledge or a more surefire way to avoid falling into the same trap again. By focusing on the progress that you have made and reminding yourself of your ultimate goals, you can overcome setbacks and stay motivated on your sugar-smart journey.

As we conclude this chapter, there is a need to emphasise the importance of embracing a sustainable approach. By shifting your mindset, practising self-compassion, building a supportive network, and navigating social situations confidently, you can maintain long-term success in reducing sugar consumption and prioritising your overall well-being.

Embracing a sugar-smart lifestyle is a continuous journey. With the strategies and tools discussed so far in this book, you can create a sustainable, balanced, and fulfilling life that supports your health and happiness.

Here's to a future filled with vitality, mindful choices, and the empowerment to live a sugar-smart lifestyle!

Chapter Nine

EMBRACING A LIFETIME OF SWEET WELLNESS

Embracing a lifetime of sweet wellness is a journey. If you expect to see positive changes in your physical health and mental well-being, then it is required that you remain consistent, committed, and willing to take steps to attain progress.

In this chapter, we will reflect on the journey towards a sugar-smart lifestyle and look ahead to the future. It is time to embrace a sweet and balanced future where you can enjoy the pleasures of life while prioritising your health and well-being. We will also explore the key principles of maintaining a sugar-smart lifestyle and offer insights to help you sustain your progress and continue to thrive.

Finding Your Balance

As you strive to lead a sugar-smart life, finding the balance that works best for you as an individual is important. In this section, we will delve into the concept of intuitive eating, listening to your body's cues, and finding the right equilibrium between indulgence and nourishment.

By embracing moderation and allowing yourself occasional treats in controlled portions, you can enjoy the sweetness of life without compromising your health. Instead of living on strict dieting rules, you can find a balance between what you eat and how you eat.

Intuitive eating emphasises trusting your inner hunger and fullness cues and freeing yourself from dieting or rigid eating rules. It promotes a more mindful and intuitive approach to nourishing oneself.

Registered dietitians Evelyn Tribole and Elyse Resch first introduced the concept of intuitive eating in their book *Intuitive Eating: A Revolutionary Program That Works*. The basic principles of intuitive eating mentioned in the book include:

- **Reject the Diet Mentality**

    Let go of the dieting mindset and the pursuit of quick-fix weight loss. Recognise that diets often lead to cyclical patterns of restriction and overeating. As the body's hunger signals intensify and feelings of deprivation grow, sustaining a strict diet becomes difficult. This can lead to episodes of overeating, where individuals consume large quantities of food, often high in calories and typically the ones that were restricted.

- **Honour Your Hunger**

  Listen to your body's cues for hunger and respond appropriately by eating when you feel hungry. Avoid ignoring or suppressing hunger signals. Give yourself unconditional permission to eat all foods without guilt or judgment. This includes allowing yourself to enjoy healthy and indulgent foods in moderation.

- **Discover the Satisfaction Factor**

  Enjoy the eating experience and savour the flavours and textures of your food. Eating should be pleasurable and satisfying. Also, pay attention to your body's signals of fullness and stop eating when you are comfortably satisfied, even if food is left on your plate.

- **Cope With Emotions Without Food**

  Find alternative ways to cope with stress, boredom, or other emotions instead of turning to food for comfort.

- **Honour Your Health**

  Make food choices that support your physical and mental health, but remember that no single meal or food choice determines your overall health.

Intuitive eating helps individuals break free from the cycle of dieting and allows them to develop a more positive and sustainable relationship with food and their bodies. However, working with a registered dietitian or healthcare professional is essential if you have specific health concerns or conditions.

Continued Education and Learning

Knowledge is a powerful tool on your journey towards a sugar-smart lifestyle. The importance of staying informed about the latest research, trends, and insights regarding sugar and nutrition cannot be overemphasised. More so, continued education empowers you to make well-informed choices, adapt to evolving scientific findings, and remain proactive in your pursuit of a balanced and healthy life.

Continuous education is vital because it helps you stay informed about the latest research and developments in various aspects of health and well-being, such as nutrition, exercise, mental health, and stress management. With this knowledge, you can make more informed and conscious choices about your sweet wellness journey, leading to better health outcomes.

Secondly, being educated about healthy living can help you identify potential risk factors and take preventive measures to avoid health issues. For example, understanding the importance of regular exercise and a balanced diet can help prevent chronic conditions like heart disease, obesity, and diabetes.

Thirdly, continuous learning creates sustainable habits. By equipping yourself with the necessary tools and resources, you are developing yourself in the process as well as creating sustainable and long-lasting healthy habits. Also, gathering necessary knowledge goes beyond short-term fad diets or temporary lifestyle changes. Instead, it promotes a holistic approach to well-being.

Gaining knowledge on your journey to a sugar-smart lifestyle helps you maintain a balanced and healthy lifestyle. By this, you become a positive role model for others, like your family members, friends, or colleagues. Your actions can inspire and motivate them to make positive changes in their lives.

Lastly, continued learning empowers you to live a long life and age gracefully. A healthy lifestyle, combined with staying mentally active through learning, can contribute to longevity and promote ageing gracefully with better cognitive function and physical health. In other words, by staying curious and inquisitive, you are bound to make positive changes in your sugar-smart lifestyle while you enjoy improved well-being and a more fulfilling life.

Mindful Living Beyond Food

Leading a sugar-smart lifestyle extends beyond food choices. It encompasses all aspects of your well-being. You need to cultivate a holistic approach to self-care by prioritising sleep, engaging in regular physical activity, managing stress, and nurturing positive relationships. Caring for your mind, body, and spirit creates a foundation of overall wellness that supports your sugar-smart journey and enhances the quality of your life.

As we discuss this section, you will better understand mindful living and incorporate practices such as meditation, stress management techniques, and self-care rituals into your daily routine.

- **Meditation**

Meditation is a fundamental practice in mindful living. It involves intentionally focusing on a particular object, thought, or activity to develop awareness and achieve mental clarity.

Various methods of meditation are breath-focused, loving-kindness, body scan, and mindfulness meditation. Consistent meditation can reduce stress, improve concentration, and foster a greater sense of inner peace and well-being.

- **Stress management techniques**

Mindful living encourages the adoption of stress management techniques to cope with the challenges of daily living. Deep breathing exercises, progressive muscle relaxation, and guided imagery are some techniques that can help reduce stress and promote relaxation.

Mindfulness-based stress reduction (MBSR) programs, which combine mindfulness meditation with stress management practices, have also been shown to be beneficial for managing stress and anxiety.

- **Self-care rituals**

Self-care is a vital aspect of mindful living, as it involves intentionally taking time to nurture and care for oneself. Self-care rituals can include engaging in activities that promote relaxation and well-being, such as taking a warm bath, nature walk, practising yoga, reading a book, or spending time with loved ones. These rituals help reduce burnout and improve overall mental and emotional health.

Inspiring Others and Creating a Ripple Effect

Embracing a sugar-smart lifestyle isn't just about you. It is about inspiring others and creating a ripple effect of positive change in their lives. Your journey towards a sugar-smart lifestyle can inspire others to make positive changes. Inspiring others entails leading by example, sharing your experiences, and offering support and encouragement to those around you. By creating a ripple effect of wellness and inspiring others to make mindful choices, you contribute to a healthier and happier community.

Every choice you make matters, and each small step towards a sugar-smart lifestyle is a step toward improved well-being and vitality. As you discover the hidden sweetness in whole foods and reduce your reliance on added sugars, you inspire your friends, family, and communities to rethink their approach to nutrition and overall health. By doing so, you are creating a ripple effect of positive change that extends far beyond yourself.

Feel free to share tips, recipes, and stories of triumph and resilience to support your tribe, friends, and colleagues every step of the way. Celebrate every milestone you accomplish, learn from challenges, and lift each person. Rest assured that those you have inspired will replicate what they have learnt from you in the lives of others and those they care about.

As we conclude this chapter, I celebrate the progress you have made on your journey toward a sugar-smart lifestyle. By now, I believe you've learnt about the impact of sugar on your health, strategies to conquer cravings, the role of physical activity, and practical tools for sustainable change. Armed with this knowledge, you have a responsibility to embrace a future that is both sweet and balanced.

May this journey inspire you to make conscious choices, nourish your body, and nurture your overall well-being. Remember that leading a sugar-smart lifestyle is not about deprivation or restriction but about finding harmony and enjoyment in your choices.

You create a foundation for a fulfilling and vibrant life by prioritising your health and embracing balance. Here's to a future where sweetness and vitality coexist and where you can thrive pursuing a sugar-smart and joyful existence.

Chapter Ten

RESOURCES FOR CONTINUED SUPPORT AND GROWTH

Welcome to the last chapter of this book. I believe it's been a wholesome journey for you from the beginning until now. Achieving holistic health and maintaining a sugar-wise lifestyle is a continuous endeavour that spans our entire life. While this book is intended to serve as a full-length resource for you, you should also consistently seek support and information to sustain the progress you've achieved through this book.

In this chapter, I will provide a compilation of invaluable resources for your continued support and growth on your sugar-wise lifestyle journey. These resources will help you uphold your commitment to being mindful of sugar consumption. Embracing a sugar-wise lifestyle extends beyond temporary actions; it involves establishing a sustainable, long-term approach to your overall well-being. The shared resources in this chapter will bridge this gap.

These resources include books, blogs, mobile apps, health professionals, and workshops.

1. **Books and Literature**

Books are an incredible resource that equip you with knowledge, ignite your imagination, and guide various facets of life. In light of this, so many books border on nutrition that will help you, just like this one in your hands. I have taken the time to curate a collection of books that delve deeply into the realms of sugar, nutrition, mindful eating, and holistic well-being. They serve as a treasure house of valuable insights that empower you to make informed decisions and cultivate a sugar-wise lifestyle.

These titles include:

- *Unsavoury Truth* by Marion Nestle

- *How Not to Die* by Michael Greger, M.D., with Gene Stone

- *Gut: The Inside Story of Our Body's Most Underrated Organ* by Giulia Enders

- *Sugar: The World Corrupted: From Slavery to Obesity* by James Walvin

- *Mindful Eating: A Guide to Rediscovering a Healthy and Joyful Relationship with Food* by Jan Chozen Bays

Each book contains actionable advice and knowledge grounded in research. I can guarantee that they will guide you towards a healthier and more harmonious life.

2. Online Communities and Websites

We live in a modern-interconnected era, and the Internet presents a wealth of invaluable resources and supportive networks that we can benefit from. In the digital realm, various platforms offer a wide array of resources for anyone interested in making wise sugar consumption choices.

Here are some websites, blogs, and online communities that serve this purpose:

The Art of Healthy Living (artofhealthyliving.com)
Well+Good (wellandgood.com)
Bites of Wellness (bitesofwellne ss.com)
Nutrition Resource Hub (health.com/nutrition)
Nutrition facts (nutritionfacts.org)

Engaging with the resources shared on these blog sites gives you the potential for a lasting sense of motivation as you continue on the sugar-wise lifestyle. Many of them are truly inspiring and will propel you to make educated decisions concerning your nutritional needs. In the same vein, joining relevant online communities and connecting with individuals who share similar health goals can help you establish a supportive network of friends online.

These networks enrich your journey and provide encouragement, solace, insights, and unity. The interesting part is that they are readily accessible online. All you have to do is research to figure out what online community is most relevant to your needs. Remember, the internet has much to offer if you can leverage it.

3. Nutritionists and Health Professionals

Nutritionists and health professionals are also highly beneficial in leading a sugar-wise lifestyle. These individuals often possess the essential education, training, and expertise to offer precise guidance. Seeking health professionals is a guaranteed strategy that helps you receive tailored medical advice distinct to your health situation.

Nutritionists and health professionals possess an in-depth understanding of how sugar impacts health. They are adept at evaluating eating patterns, preferences, and health aspirations. Thus, they are qualified to offer suggestions that will help you make informed decisions regarding your health. This may include designing a wholesome meal plan that serves your specific nutritional needs, proposing healthier substitutes, or devising strategies you can use holistically to conquer sugar cravings.

They are also capable of addressing your health concerns, for instance, if you're a diabetic patient or have challenges with obesity. Health professionals can supply evidence-based information that will assist you in making knowledgeable decisions related to your dietary and life habits.

The interesting part is that you can get continuous support from nutritionists and healthcare professionals because they oversee your progress closely, modify your strategies, and encourage you toward a healthier lifestyle. This consistent support can prove indispensable in upholding your motivation and achieving your health goals.

4. Mobile Apps and Tools

We're in the digital era, and the widespread availability of smartphones and devices has transformed how we engage with life and other people. This does not exclude our dietary behaviours and general well-being. Imagine scrolling through Instagram, and an ad from a brewing company keeps popping up on your screen. You naturally begin to think about consuming beer and enjoy the great feeling the ad has reinforced in your mind. Another instance is when you come in touch with different ideologies spanning the various aspects of life through Twitter by tweeting and retweeting others' posts. And isn't food/nutrition one important aspect of human life?

The good part is that these technologies can help you lead a better lifestyle if you use them wisely. With the advent of the internet came the development of web and mobile applications catering to the specific needs of a target audience. Nowadays, it is easy to find mobile applications that serve as useful resources for individuals who aim to embrace a lifestyle conscious of sugar consumption.

There are different categories of apps, as some concentrate fully on meal planning. Others help you monitor your diet, and a few help you assess the sugar content in a particular product by enabling you to scan its barcode just before consumption. Some apps have mindfulness exercises and techniques that advocate a mindful approach to eating. These practices encourage users to relish each bite and be more attuned to their hunger and fullness signals, thereby fostering a healthier relationship with food.

Another category of apps is those that include exercise monitoring features that help you stay consistent with your fitness regimen while monitoring your progress in real time. This fitness integration complements your sugar consumption journey, helping you attain a holistic lifestyle that balances your dietary choices with your physical fitness.

If used effectively, these mobile apps and tools can help you stay organised, monitor your progress, and stay accountable to your goals. Such apps include PlateJoy, Lose It!, Eat This Much, BigOven, etc. You can search them out at your leisure. There is a plethora of other apps you can find online that may also suit your needs.

5. **Continuing Education and Workshops**

Continued education and attending workshops provide opportunities for growth and learning. Attending seminars, workshops, and conferences focused on nutrition, mindfulness, and overall well-being can be an added advantage to your journey toward a sugar-wise lifestyle. These events offer opportunities to expand your knowledge, connect with like-minded individuals, and gain new perspectives on leading a sugar-smart lifestyle.

Remember that having a room full of people pursuing the same goals as you can serve as a huge morale booster as you embark on this journey to wise sugar consumption, mindful eating, and a healthy lifestyle.

As I conclude this chapter, let me remind you that you are not alone in this pursuit of wellness. Numerous resources are available to support and guide you on your path to balance, health, and fulfilment. By utilising those shared in this chapter, engaging with supportive communities, and continuing your personal growth, you can sustain your progress and thrive in your commitment to a sugar-wise lifestyle.

May you continuously embrace the ongoing nature of this journey and remain open to learning, evolving, and supporting others along the way.

Here's to a future filled with knowledge, connection, and empowerment as you, countless others, and I navigate the path toward optimal well-being and a sugar-wise life together!

CONCLUSION

This book has been a long journey towards a more vibrant living by reducing sugar intake. So far, you have learnt to listen to your body's whispers, honouring its requirements while managing your desires with innovative alternatives. You have discovered the rhythm of your body by prioritising physical activity, finding joy in movement, and embracing vitality in every step.

Throughout this journey, you have discovered that leading a sugar-smart lifestyle is not about deprivation or strict rules but about finding balance, making informed choices, and nurturing your overall well-being.

By reducing your sugar intake, you have learnt to take a proactive step towards improving your health and vitality. You have learnt to listen to your body, honour your cravings, and find alternative ways to satisfy your sweet tooth. You have embraced the power of mindful eating, regular physical activity, and prioritising self-care as essential components of a well-rounded and fulfilling life. Throughout this journey, you have recognised the importance of support and community.

You have also discovered the value of connecting with like-minded individuals, seeking professional guidance, and sharing your experiences to inspire others. By fostering a sense of support, accountability, and understanding, you will find the motivation to continue thriving on your sugar-smart path.

As I conclude this book, I want to remind you that the journey towards a sugar-smart lifestyle is not a one-time endeavour. It is a lifelong commitment to your well-being, a continuous growth process, and an opportunity for personal transformation.

You will encounter challenges, setbacks, and moments of temptation along the way. However, armed with the knowledge and tools explored in this book, you can overcome these obstacles and embrace a life filled with sweet wellness.

May this journey remind you that you can take control of your health and make choices that align with your values and aspirations.

Each day is an opportunity to prioritise your well-being, nourish your body, and savour life's sweetness. As you move forward with confidence, compassion, and a commitment to leading a sugar-smart lifestyle that nurtures your health and happiness, I hope you achieve balance, feel empowered, and enjoy sweet wellness.

Cheers!

SWEET WELLNESS

85

ONEN JOSHUA

SWEET WELLNESS